# WE JUST SAID

# NO!

# TREATING ADHD WITHOUT MEDICATION

# A STEP-BY-STEP GUIDE TO INCREASING FOCUS AND IMPROVING MOOD

## BY

## Kasey Phillips Brown, LCSW

This book contains steps we took to prevent our son from being prescribed psychotropic medication. This is not a medical book and no medical interventions are given. Please consult with your pediatrician before implementing any of the interventions listed.

www.newperspectivesprograms.com
Printed in the United States of America
First Printing: April 2017
www.Bookbaby.com
ISBN- 978-1-54390-042-2

# Table of Contents

# Introduction

When my son was around 2 yrs. old I noticed, he was very hyper and would run around a lot. Because I have been hyper all of my life and I have the ability to do 4-5 things at one time, I knew he could possibly have symptoms of Attention Deficit Hyperactivity Disorder (ADHD) like me. However, since I am a Licensed Clinical Social Worker and I knew that at that time, ADHD couldn't be diagnosed until after age 5, I just began to watch him more closely.

Around the same time that I noticed his hyperactivity one of my Occupational Therapy (OT) friends was concerned about the fact that he would always fall down while running. She recommended that I get him assessed by the local Regional Center, which assesses children and sometimes adults for developmental disabilities. An O.T. came to our home to evaluate him. A few weeks later we received a report that stated that there were no concerns. I continued to observe him.

I enrolled him in an emergent learning preschool program that was connected to a college. It was a training lab for teachers. The curriculum focused on learning through play and self-expression. Even with the freedom of that environment, it was hard for him to follow directions. He would often run from thing to thing and it was difficult for him to focus on one activity for an extended amount of time. We had lots of parent teacher conferences to try to assist him in completing tasks. There were many tearful nights as I stayed awake worrying about him starting kindergarten in a couple of years and stressing about how he was going to adjust to an environment that required more structure.

When he started kindergarten the teacher's only concern was that he had a difficult time holding his pencil and learning how to write. I again reached out to my O.T. friends and they provided me with some occupational therapy techniques to help him increase his fine motor skills.

First grade is when the teacher had deeper concerns and believed that additional interventions were needed in order for our child to succeed academically. He requested we have a SST meeting (Student Study Team or Student Success Team) that includes the principal, teachers and school psychologist to address the challenges my son was facing daily in the classroom.

During the meeting, I was very clear with the different teachers, school psychologist and the principal and my husband that I was not interested in using medication to address his ADHD symptoms. Due to my profession, I am very much aware of the criteria for ADHD and I felt that my son had the symptoms that met the criteria. I did not want my child to be tested by the school and I did not want any diagnosis to be documented in his school records. I also did not want an Individualized Educational Plan (IEP) as I have seen how so many children get these plans and the schools don't follow through with the interventions and now you have a kid with a mental health diagnosis, in special education classes and they are still doing poorly in school. Honestly, if I felt that my son was going to get a thorough treatment plan and that the school would stick to the plan and give him all the extra services that he needed and in the end when he became an adult the special education services and diagnosis would not be a hindrance to his success, I may have gone that route. But I didn't have faith in the system.

I was extremely discouraged. I prayed then remembered our Clark Atlanta University motto, *Find a Way or Make One*. I began to research options and create a plan that would allow my son to have a functioning life without having him be prescribed psychotropic medication or a diagnosis at such an early age. I had a friend who had been diagnosed with multiple sclerosis and she had used holistic practitioners in her treatment. I asked her for recommendations on what I could do for my son and she suggested a chiropractor and/or dietary changes. I went on social media and asked around to see if anyone knew of a chiropractor that specializes in working with young children. Someone pointed me in the direction of a chiropractor in Pasadena. As I was researching Dr. Darrick Sahara, D.C. I sent his information to my best friend/my son's godmother and to my manager/friend. I found out that my best friend had gone to chiropractic school with him and my manager had gone to high school with him. Both of them love me and want what's best for my son. I trust them and knowing they knew him, made me feel a lot more comfortable. From the first day, we started to work with him I started to feel relief. It was great to hear someone talk to me about natural ways to deal with these symptoms. For the first time in years I began to feel like there was light at the end of this often-daunting tunnel. I could breathe again.

*Call Dr. Hekedman*

Dr. Sahara performed a thorough examination of my son's physiology and functioning, a health history, and general health examination, followed by an Applied Kinesiology (AK) examination. He adjusted my son's vertebrae and administered a "EB" therapy cleanse detox made of water and sea salt to eliminate from his body the toxins from the environment and the food that he had been eating. He prescribed a serious diet change, supplements and physical activity. We were so happy with the results we saw, that we had our younger son receive treatment as well. He does not have ADHD symptoms but has benefitted from overall good health and his moodiness has decreased.

We started this non-medication program in 2009 the summer before my son went to 2nd grade. It has been a long tough road. However, during the most recent examinations of his body movement and muscle strength, his chiropractor has observed a definite decrease in his hyperactivity and a very noticeable increase in his maturity and ability to focus. Last year he finished off the year with the best grades he has ever had. This past semester has been more difficult and his grades are suffering even though he can verbally explain the material. He states that when he starts a test his first thought is that he is going to fail. Normally, he does better the second semester as he learns what's expected of him. But it is still frustrating to see such a bright young man receive below average grades. Our goal is for his grades to improve as the years go on and as we make adjustments at home and continue to advocate for him at school. If necessary, we will even change schools to make sure our child has the best learning environment to meet his needs. I actually think he would benefit from a smaller classroom setting and I'm strongly considering a partial home school program that's nearby our home.

This has been the most difficult struggle of my life. It has been stressful and heartbreaking for us as parents to see our child trying to be seen as "normal". We have started the 2nd semester of 8th grade and are looking forward to success and striving for another medication-free year. It's been hard but worth it.

It's important to know that this book contains information and interventions that can be used with any child, not just a child who has ADHD symptoms. Also, don't be discouraged if you didn't try some of the interventions earlier. It's never too late to make a new start. I also understand that changing your child's lifestyle might feel scary and overwhelming but you can do it. You may have to be very tough in the beginning but they will get use to it. Remember you are not alone. This book was written to let you know the steps we took and the challenges we went through to naturally treat our son's ADHD symptoms. This is our journey.

# NOTES

Take Jules 2 Chiropractor

# What is ADHD?

ADHD symptoms can be present in both children and adults. It's when a person seems to be in a constant state of movement and thought. They run around and talk non-stop. They report that they have "lots of stuff on their mind" or it's observed that they seem to be day dreaming a lot or their mind is elsewhere. They might also act immediately without thinking.

Now this may sound like normal behavior for most people. It becomes a problem when it prevents someone from living a fulfilling life. For example, they can't get good grades in school because they can't focus in class. Or they can't get promoted at work because they can't keep up with their workload or constantly interrupt co-workers by blurting out their thoughts. It may cause problems with their spouse because they are forgetful or are messy or make impulsive decisions without consulting.

# NOTES

# ADHD Symptoms

To be diagnosed with ADHD a person 16 and younger must have 6 of the 9 symptoms for 6 months from the two areas below. If 17 or older they only need to have 5:

## Lack of Focus

Difficult time focusing on homework or on work task or household chores. _____

Makes a simple mistake because they didn't pay attention to the instructions that were given. _____

Need to be told something more than one time to make sure they understand the instructions completely. It may look like they're not listening when they are being spoken to. They look like they are daydreaming. _____

May not finish tasks or assignments. ____

Dis-organized school desk, workspace or home. Messy school folders, office files and or dressers at home. _____

Avoids school work that requires lots of steps like math word problems or tasks at work where there are lots of steps. _____

Loses things like homework, pens, papers or misplaces documents at work. _____

Forgets writing down class assignments, appointments. _____

Easily distracted when things are going on around them. _____

**Hyperactive Behavior/Impulsive 6 or more symptoms for at least 6 months**

Hard time sitting still i.e., moving around, swinging their feet, tapping their fingers. _____

Finds it difficult to remain seated. _____

Runs around on the playground more than other kids their age, climb on the desk at school or furniture in the home. _____

Finds it difficult to sit quietly and read a book, do a puzzle, play with toys or meditate. _____

Always moving and going. _____

Talks constantly. _____

## Impulsive Behavior

Hard time waiting their turn in their classrooms, playing games or in work meetings. _____

Cuts others off while they are talking. _____

Blurts out answers before the question has been asked. _____

# NOTES

# Important Reminder

To be diagnosed with ADHD a person must display the symptoms between the ages of 5 and 12yrs old. Anyone 4 or younger cannot be diagnosed with ADHD.

You can only be diagnosed with ADHD if the person has the symptoms in at least 2 places. Therefore, they would need to display symptoms at home and at school or at home and at work or at school and at work. If someone can sit quietly at home and focus on chores but cannot at school, then it may be a structure or school issue. There may be distractions in the class or lack of structure. If someone can pay attention in class, remember assignments and not interrupt peers or teachers but is running all over their home, jumping on furniture and not following directions at home, it may be a discipline or other issue in the home.

# NOTES

# Differential Diagnosis

Other disorders that look like ADHD:

**PTSD**-Person may have a difficult time concentrating.

**Depression**-Person may have a difficult time concentrating or paying attention, they may fidget (psychomotor agitation), and have a hard time completing task (low motivation).

**Sensory Integration Issues** -Person may move around a lot (fidget), have emotional dysregulation (easily upset), have body boundary issues (bumping into others).

***PTSD and Depression can be assessed by a Clinical Social Worker, Marriage and Family Therapist, Psychologist or other mental health professional. Sensory Integration Issues can be assessed by an Occupational Therapist.

# NOTES

# Additional Disorders

Sometimes children with ADHD become so frustrated by the barriers they face at home and at school and at all the negative feedback they receive, that they begin to "act out". The behaviors and or feelings can result in a child having ADHD and Persistent Depressive Disorder or ADHD and Oppositional Defiant Disorder.

I am not including this to create more stress or increase feelings of sadness. I am mentioning this because it's important to know that this can happen and by following some of the techniques I discuss in this book you may be able to prevent additional behavioral and emotional issues and in turn prevent a secondary diagnosis for your child.

# NOTES

# O.T. Assessment

If you think your child has ADHD one of the first things you should do is have him assessed by an Occupational Therapist (O.T.). This assessment will determine if there is a certain skill set or deficiency in communication, gross motor, personal and social interactions, problem solving and in fine motor skills.

We scheduled an OT assessment for our son when he was a toddler to assess if he was having other issues that we were not aware of. ADHD is a common misdiagnosis for someone who may actually have a Sensory Integration Disorder. The assessment would take place in your home, in a school or in a clinic. It could consist of the O.T. observing your child's gross and fine motor skills, behavior and movement as well as your child's response to stimuli.

You can find an O.T. in your area through your local hospital, your child's school or through American Occupational Therapy Association (AOTA) www.aota.org

# NOTES

# Chiropractic

Working with our son's chiropractor, Dr. Darrick Sahara DC, was one of the best decisions we made. He was able to explain how the starches our son was eating (breads, potatoes, rice, pizza, noodles) don't process well in his liver; therefore, there is an overabundance of sugar left, which causes bloating in the liver that results in hyperactivity. In my younger son those foods don't process well in his gallbladder which causes him to be more emotional, resulting in him being extremely emotional.

Their chiropractor performs an adjustment of the spine then does a foot detox which removes toxins from the body caused by food and the environment. His treatment also includes kinesiology (the study of non-human/human movement). Initially he treated them every two weeks. Now they go every 2-3 months as needed or when I can remember to make the appointments.

# NOTES

# Dietary Plan

Per our chiropractor's instruction we immediately changed their diets to a protein and vegetable diet. There is no starch allowed although they can have minimal breading on some foods. The hardest challenge was that my son considers himself to be a vegetarian although he loves bacon. It was extremely difficult to get him to try different meat dishes. At first, we implemented the diet change daily but as the Chiropractor noticed that their bodies were more balanced we only did it Mon-Fri morning. Friday night through Sunday they could have their pizza and other birthday party/weekend foods.

It was very difficult to supervise his eating while at school. He had a little friend who would often give him pizza and other food. We tried to monitor it but it was nearly impossible, so we had to make sure we stayed consistent during weekday breakfast, snacks and dinner.

# NOTES

- Turkey Hot dogs
- chicken
- less mac & cheese
- Spinach
- Kale
- less Sugars/sweets
- Change the snacks mom gives them.
- Veggie burgers
- chili
- Make sure they help cook.

# Protein

Protein is the main staple of his diet. He has meat for breakfast, lunch and dinner. The biggest obstacle we faced is the fact that my son considers himself to be a vegetarian. I would normally support this mindset but he eats bacon, pepperoni, chicken nuggets and turkey. Therefore, he is a selective vegetarian so I encouraged him to diversify his pallet some. However, since bacon is by far his favorite food we centered his breakfast and lunch around it.

Little by little I would try different types of protein. It would really just depend on his taste buds. I think a lot of it is that he doesn't like the texture of meat. Again, his dislike of most meat resulted in him eating a lot of the same things each day.

We couldn't substitute peanuts or nuts because he was allergic. We tried some bean recipes but he didn't really like beans either.

# NOTES

# Water

Water is such an essential part of a having a healthy and balanced body. In lieu of orange juice or milk at breakfast we give our children water. They also use to take water to school for snack and or lunch. This dietary change eliminated milk, juice, soda or any other drinks. On weekends, we allowed some other drinks but it was considered a special treat.

Often people (not just kids) will think that they are hungry when really, they are just dehydrated. We made sure he had several glasses of water a day. This also helped create very regular bowel movements.

As they got older it was extremely difficult to control their water intake at school. Also at home if juice or sodas were brought into the home they would sneak them. It's best to have everyone in the home drinking the same things if possible. I've had to ask my husband to hide his juice in our room.

# NOTES

more water
water w/breakfast

# Vegetables

Believe it or not this was the easiest part of the lifestyle change. Our son loves vegetables. That made it very easy to incorporate them into every one of his daily meals. He likes almost every vegetable so we had plenty to choose from. However, as with most kids they go through their "picky" phase and when this happened we would simply keep it simple like the bacon and give him the vegetable he liked the most, over and over again.

There were days and weeks when he would have broccoli for breakfast and dinner. The vegetables we used the most were broccoli, peas, spinach and zucchini. Although peas, zucchini and squash are considered starchy vegetables, we did make those but just not as much.

I really wanted to plant a garden full of my own vegetables but something always came up and I never found the time. It still remains one of my goals. I would have the boys maintain it.

# NOTES

Can have veeggees
w/breakfast

# Fruit

Although fruit contains natural sugar, we followed our chiropractor's instruction and limited his fruit intake to twice a day as a snack. We would give him a snack after school and before dinner. The fruit that we used for snack were apples as he seemed to like those the most. According to their chiropractor our kids were able to have almost any fruit except for bananas. When I asked the chiropractor about giving the boys fruit smoothies he made it clear that he didn't feel like it was the best way for them to get their nutrition. His exact words were, "Kids need to use their teeth."

We didn't make a large effort to buy organic fruit or go to Farmer's markets. Not because we had an issue with it, we just didn't have a lot of time so we just bought fruit from our local grocery store. And like the vegetables the goal was always to grow our own fruit.

# NOTES

# Supplements

Initially we tried to implement the supplements that the chiropractor recommended, like fish oil, cod liver oil, Omega 3s and other sprays and vitamins. After each exam, he would let us know the supplement at that time that would best create optimal health. We understood that we would see quicker and better results if we gave them supplements but it was a constant fight to get the kids to swallow them and it was expensive to keep buying them when they would not take them. So, we stopped the supplements. Now that they are older I am strongly considering putting supplements back into their routine as they are older and now better able to understand the benefits of the them.

# NOTES

# Eliminating Starch

This was one of the most difficult parts of changing my son's lifestyle. His favorite foods are pizza, rice, noodles, waffles, pancakes, potatoes and bread. He was not happy at all about not being able to eat those foods. We initially went cold turkey and removed those foods from his diet for about two months. There was a lot of complaining and crying but he eventually complied. Once the chiropractor began to notice an increase in his muscle strength, and body balance we began to allow some of these things on the weekend.

There are also some vegetables and fruits that are high in starch so we removed those from the diets too.

We changed my younger son's diet too. A low starch diet is also extremely helpful in preventing mood swings, grumpiness and temper tantrums.

# NOTES

# Eliminating Sugar

This was also a very difficult task. We removed all foods that have sugar from his diet for two months except for apples. Although we did not often give him candy or sweets, they were completely removed from his diet. No candy, soda, cookies, or other sticky treats. Again, once he had an examination by the chiropractor that showed he was balanced and his focus had improved we allowed sugary treats during special occasions.

It is surprising how many items that we consume have high sugar levels. When reading labels, look for the words: glucose, crystal dextrose, corn syrup, cane juice, molasses, fructose, lactose and maltose.

# NOTES

# Eliminating Dairy

We removed dairy by no longer having cereal or dishes that contain cheese. We previously would give him 2% milk but stopped giving that as well during the week. Later we brought those dishes back during the weekend along with ice cream.

One of the benefits of removing dairy was that our children never again had runny or stuffy noses. There was not a lot of coughing or sneezing at all. True story, about 2 years ago, I was startled by hearing what sounded like someone blowing their nose in the back seat. I was so surprised by the sound and quickly questioned the boys. It turned out it was the car. But that showed me how rarely I hear my boys blow their noses.

# NOTES

# Sample Meals
## BREAKFAST

Bacon and broccoli

Scrambled eggs with zucchini with bacon

Sausage and eggs and string beans

Mixed veggies with hot dogs (no bun)

Vegetable, tomato, lentil soup

Tilapia and Broccoli

Salmon and mixed vegetables

Hamburger patty and broccoli

Sautéed Kale and tomato omelet

Chorizo and beans

Fast food restaurant-Bacon, sausage, eggs

# NOTES

# LUNCH

Lunch was difficult because it was hard to supervise him at school and keep vegetables warm. We basically sent him with bacon and or pineapples. He would eat a snack when he got home from school. But lunch should be any meat and vegetable combo. Most of the choices below can be found at a fast food restaurant if you are in a hurry.

Salad

Hamburger, lettuce tomato (no bun)

Chicken nuggets

Chicken strips

Hot dog (no bun)

Hot wings

Lettuce wraps with lunch meat inside

# NOTES

# DINNER

Chicken nuggets and salad

Tacos with lettuce shells (Kale chip or Romaine) *Make tacos w/ kids*

Spaghetti Squash with meatballs

Baked chicken with pinto beans

Pork chops and peas

Turkey sausage and cabbage

Ribs and greens

Steak and spinach

Noodles (made of zucchini) with stir-fry vegetables and Shrimp

Pot roast and string beans

Meat loaf and salad

# NOTES

# Physical Activity

We put him in taekwondo (Any martial art would be fine), basketball, baseball, swimming or whatever sport was going on at the time. We made sure that after school he had some type of outlet to expend his extra energy. We played Wii Fit, Just Dance 3, The Michael Jackson Experience and any other video game that got him to move his body. Sometimes we would just go to the park and run around.

Most recently he played football which was difficult because at 13 years old he was new to the game and didn't know a lot of the terminology. It was hard for him to pick up the plays as he had never heard of most of the terms before. Also, he is a visual learner and he had a hard time following instructions that were being yelled out in a noisy huddle. However, his coach thought he was a quick learner and did a good job. He wants to play again.

# NOTES

# Naps

Kids are never too old for a nap. We have him take a nap after school each day. He can either have a snack then take a nap or take a nap then wake up and have a snack. It is important that the nap is neither too short nor too long because if it is the child could wake up extremely cranky. He is currently 13 years old and taking a nap remains part of his routine.

I realize that kids will often complain and start kicking and screaming that they are not tired but believe me, they are tired. Initially if you can, try to lie down with them. Beware, you may end up taking a nap too. I can't tell you how many good moments of sleep I ended up getting by climbing in bed with them. Glad I did it because I really did need the rest.

One good thing is that as he got older (12-13) I didn't have to make him take a nap anymore. He was usually exhausted from having to wake so early for school and being gone all day, he was happy to take a nap when he got home.

# NOTES

# Bedtime

He already had a consistent bedtime but we continued to implement it.

Under 7 years old bedtime was 7:00pm

8-9 years old bedtime – 8:00pm

10 years old and up- 9pm

Just like with the dietary changes, the Bedtime schedule was not used every day. Sunday through Thursday they had a specific bedtime and Fri and Sat they could stay up a little later.

Having a scheduled bedtime also allowed for my husband and I to have more downtime at night. It's nice to have some peace and quiet after a long day.

# NOTES

# Daily Schedule

*Snack*

*Physical Activity*

*Nap (easier to focus on homework when rested)*

**(NOTE: Snack, Physical activity or Nap can be in any order)**

*Homework*

*Chores*

*Extracurricular activity (piano or another class)*

*Read a book*

*Night time hygiene routine/Bedtime*

It was sometimes difficult to maintain this daily schedule due to organized sports and activities like (school plays, rehearsals, tutoring, chess, etc.) work commitments and just life in general. We did our best to stick to the schedule as much as possible.

# NOTES

# Math Coach

A math coach and math tutor can become a large additional expense for a family. If a private tutor doesn't fit into your budget, you can ask the teacher at your child's school for any free tutoring services at their school. You can also check your local library, afterschool programs, parks and community centers. There are also on-line tutoring programs.

We initially enlisted a professional math coach who has experience teaching teachers how to teach math. The math coach's focus was to assist my son with becoming familiar with math in a low stress fun environment. She provided a great foundation and engaged him in activities that introduced him to math concepts without him realizing it. We enjoyed working with her but it was difficult traveling in the middle of the week to her home that was not close to our home.

# Math Tutor

Although a math coach was no longer feasible we still needed to have someone assist our son with a subject that caused him a great deal of frustration and that was impacting his self-esteem. It also caused a lot of frustration and stress in the home. We found a math tutor who came to the house twice a week. Although we liked the tutor we noticed that our son became very comfortable and began to see her as a family member. He would joke around and not listen or pay attention as much. We eventually hired another math tutor that not only did one on one weekly sessions but provided a "fun math group" for my son and his two close friends. This "fun math group" provides an opportunity for my son to have a weekly fun experience that makes math enjoyable.

We were also able to make an arrangement with his math teacher to allow him to turn in his homework every other day so that the tutor could help him with his math homework instead of us. It was causing a great deal of stress in our house when we did math with him. This arrangement worked out well for all involved. He had a very successful year in math (compared to his previous years) and he was able to raise his grades in his primary math class and his supplemental math class, this past semester.

This semester has been extremely stressful and challenging for him. According to the tutor he understands the work but gets frustrated quickly if he doesn't get it and gives up. This is truly not my son's nature. He is a very determined person. This is the kid who taught himself how to roller skate at his kindergarten field trip because he kept falling and he looked around and saw all of his classmates rolling along. Again, this is another situation where there is a big difference between academics and his normal life. If this was a line in a play that he couldn't remember he would not stop until he knew it inside and out. At this time we are trying to figure out if we need a new tutor or do we need to explore his test anxiety.

# NOTES

# Technology

In order to leave room for reading, homework, chores, physical activity and general downtime, we limited technology in our house (television, video games, telephones) to Friday afternoon through Sunday evening. Initially there was some complaining but eventually it became a part of the family culture and they became use to it. This also helped when disciplining them as technology use was used as a reward for when they followed household rules, instructions and expectations. As they got older restricting technology became more difficult because their phones became a larger part of their life. They only got phones last year because someone else would be picking them up from school but they quickly became their life line to their friends and the rest of the world. We remained firm and they are only to use the phone on the weekend. This is difficult and harder to enforce when others are watching them.

# NOTES

# Discipline

It is imperative that a child with ADHD symptoms receives discipline and structure. We started off trying time-outs and "the naughty corner" and behavior charts. I could never remember to put the stickers on the charts or give them the rewards when they earned enough stickers, therefore we decided that the best form of discipline for our son was "Thumbs Up/Thumbs Down". It's a pretty simple concept that only needs a thumb to make it work.

My child would start off the day with my thumb pointing up to the 12 o'clock mark. If he was doing something that was not appropriate, I would simply look at him, take my thumb and start to point it counter clock wise toward the 10'oclock mark. If it even got anywhere near where 9 o'clock might be, my child would freak out and beg for a chance to get the thumb back straight up to the 12 o'clock mark.

If he got a thumb down that meant no technology on Friday night and if his behavior kept getting worse, no technology for the entire weekend. This seemed to be the worst punishment ever and he would often do his best to keep a thumb up.

# NOTES

_____

_____

_____

_____

_____

_____

_____

_____

_____

_____

_____

_____

# Behavior issues

Sometimes children with ADHD symptoms get frustrated because they either missed the assignment or don't understand it. They began to talk to their neighbors or make jokes to make their friends laugh or do anything to cover up that they are lost or to get some type of attention. We made it very clear to our son that there were not going to be any behavior issues in class. Whatever the teacher's behavior chart was, he was expected to get the highest level. We were firm with this requirement. In elementary the majority of his daily marks were high, with only a few "average" remarks when there was a substitute teacher who wasn't aware of my son's needs. With the pressures to fit in this got a little harder in middle school. We just continued to express the importance of him thinking before he acts and maintained close communication with the school. It feels good that the teachers continue to report he is a pleasure to have in class.

# NOTES

# O.T. Lap Pad

Our son was fidgeting around in his classroom seat so much that he was falling out of his chair. I did some research and found a lap pad for his age range at www.therapyshoppe.com. The lap pad is a piece of material wrapped around some weights and zipped up. It looks like a small blanket that can be draped over their lap. The lap pad is used to apply pressure and it calms the client down. I took it to the school and explained to the teacher that he was to keep the pad on his lap. After he started using this he was sitting up straight within a day or two. I eventually saw his teacher at the school reading night and she stated," Hey! Did I tell you that he's no longer using the pad? After the first few days he started to sit up straight and he stopped the fidgeting. It got to the point where he no longer needed it so I let other students use it."

**Important note:** An occupational therapist informed me that an OT assessment should be done prior to giving a child a lap pad as it could be detrimental to some children's muscles and cause them to become lethargic in class.

# NOTES

_____

_____

_____

_____

_____

_____

_____

_____

_____

_____

_____

_____

_____

_____

_____

_____

_____

_____

# Initiating Conferences

We never waited for the teachers to schedule the parent teacher conferences, which were usually held about 6-8 weeks into the school year. We felt that was too long to wait to inform the teachers of our son's needs. On the first day of school we scheduled a conference with the teacher for the following week. In that meeting, we explained that our son benefits from sitting in the front of the class, that he has a special diet, gets chiropractic treatment, takes supplements, engages in physical activities and takes daily naps. We also explained the "Thumbs up/Thumbs down" technique. This provided consistency at home and at school. When he started middle school, I created a standard letter that contained all the important information above and emailed them to each teacher. I noticed that if we didn't give the information the first day he quickly got overlooked and fell behind because he wasn't a behavior problem.

# NOTES

# Advocating at school meetings

The school meetings were extremely overwhelming for me. I had all these thoughts in my mind and I would be holding back tears feeling like no one understood what I was going through. They all saw our son one way but I saw him a different way. I saw his light. To me it was the school system that was broken not our child. Forty years ago, if I couldn't focus or had difficulty not blurting out answers, teachers helped me learn at my own pace or re-directed me. But now because in most schools there are a limited number of teachers' aides and overcrowded classes, almost any child who lacks focus and who is considered highly extroverted is viewed as the problem. I have a strong personality, which made it easy for me to speak up in these school meetings. Looking back, I am glad I stood my ground. There were times when everyone seemed to be thinking medication and getting an IEP was the only route. However, I didn't think that those interventions would be the most beneficial for my son and I was determined to help everyone else see it too. I would ask the teachers, "What is the one thing he needs to succeed?" They would say, "Just a little more time to take his test and a quiet space." That isn't enough of a reason to prescribe medication. I explained my concerns to the school, they cooperated and allowed him the extra time to take test, and turn in class and homework assignments.

## NOTES

_____

_____

_____

_____

_____

_____

_____

_____

# Pressure to use Psychotropic Meds

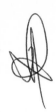

One major issue I had was that whenever we met with the teachers they would always mention that their children had been diagnosed with ADHD and that they chose to medicate them. I'm sure they thought they were being helpful with that information but honestly it would just anger me. That was the decision they made for their children but I had made a different decision. They may have been trying to decrease any stigmas attached or any anxiety that they thought we may have had regarding medication, but it just made me frustrated. With each new teacher, we met I was very clear that I wanted to manage his symptoms naturally, and thoroughly explained that medication was not an option for us. If he wants to use medication when he turns 18 that will be his decision.

# NOTES

# Self-esteem

One of the hardest things about having a child who has ADHD symptoms is watching how their self-esteem is impacted. To meet the criteria for ADHD you must display the symptoms in two different environments. That's two places where they may be getting negative feedback. Or as I like to say, that's two places where they are "getting on people's nerves". Often children with ADHD symptoms suffer with low grades. They see friends getting answers right and may become frustrated when they see siblings doing well. It hurts to hear your child say, "I'm not smart." Or to know they don't participate because they don't want to be laughed at. Public speaking is my son's gift so it's very frustrating and sad to hear all of his current teachers describe him as shy. He's not. He will make an excellent speech in any environment, at any time, about any topic. He won the cake-decorating contest in cub scouts by doing an impromptu speech about friendship and connecting it to the decorations he used. He was one of the key speakers at his 6th grade promotion and his speech received a standing ovation. We allow him to lead family grace in our immediate household and when we have or attend large family/community gatherings. In order to increase his self-esteem, we made it a point to cater to his strengths, encourage his talents and put him in situations where he was able to excel. We encouraged him to enter the church essay/speech contest (he won). We then continued to put him into situations where he had the opportunity to get positive feedback. He sang/danced in talent shows and he acted in plays. Since he was 5 he has aspired to be a marine biologist so we recently interviewed and were accepted into the USA's 2nd largest Aquarium family volunteer program. He will be educating visitors about marine life.

Also, for the 3rd year in a row he won 1st place in his school's National PTA Reflections contest. In 6th grade he wrote a song and in 7th grade he wrote a poem.

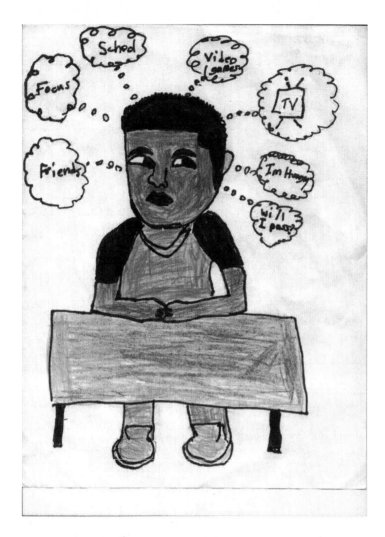

This year in 8th grade, Kaleb again won 1st place. The theme was "My Story". These are the thoughts he has in class. In the bottom cloud on the right he wrote "Will I pass?" That's his daily concern.

# NOTES

# Extra Benefits

**NO CAVITIES**- Neither of my children have had cavities. I think it has a lot to do with the fact that they drink very little sugary drinks (soda, juice) and have very little direct sugar in other food. Our sons did not even know that people put sugar on cereal until 2015. That is HILARIOUS because as a child I would put sugar on Frosted Flakes!!!

**PERFECT ATTENDANCE**- Both kids basically get perfect attendance every year. My son with the ADHD symptoms usually gets sick two days a year (pink eye or a cold) but for the most part they rarely get sick or miss school.

**ASTHMA**- He was previously diagnosed with mild asthma. Once we started this lifestyle change he did not have any more asthma attacks.

**ECZEMA**- When our sons were born they had eczema. Now their skin is completely clear. No rash like flare ups.

# NOTES

# Getting on the same page with:
## PARTNER

Although you and your partner both love your child, you may have different ways to approach this issue. It is important that you spend lots of time communicating your feelings and wants for your child. Often partners have different backgrounds and may think differently about medication, holistic approaches or even dietary changes. It's extremely important not to assume that your partner is going to just want to go along with whatever you decide. I strongly suggest regular discussions about how each partner was raised and what were their family values when it came to food, health and medicine. The most important thing is that you educate each other and remember that everything you are doing will be for the overall good health of your child.

# KIDS

Getting the kids on board may be a challenge. Again, I have a strong personality so I was very clear that we were going to make a lifestyle change to better our quality of life and live a healthier more organized life. There was no choice. Initially there were some frustration but they eventually got on board and there were no more complaints. Did they sometimes sneak food that they weren't supposed to have during the week? Yes. But that's normal and wasn't that often.

One way that I got them on the same page when it comes to school issues and making the school year smoother, is we started doing family school goals in August of each year. This year mine was to check backpacks. My husband's was to help with school projects. The younger son's goal was to give papers that needed to be signed, the night before, not the morning of and Kaleb's was to write down assignments before leaving class. We review the goals in January and discuss any barriers and see if the goals were met. We would then evaluate the goals at the end of the school year in June.

# FAMILY

It is also essential to make sure that your family is educated and aware of the new changes that you are implementing in your child's life. Family members often babysit and spend large amounts of time with your children. It's important that they know what to feed your child, how much technology time you allow, their nap schedule and so on. In some families, what other relatives think means a lot and it's hard when you are making decisions that are not within the cultural norms.

# FRIENDS

Friends who don't agree with the holistic approach can also add to your stress. I

ignored any disapproving look.
comments and explained that this wa
way my husband and I decided to ha.
this situation. Eventually they began to see
how effective it was and there was no
longer a need to have to explain myself or
the choices that we made for our children
and our friends became a major support.

# TEACHERS

I would also be proactive in encouraging
teachers to work with one another and
share their interventions. Once I was
talking to his 3rd grade teacher on the
playground and I saw his 2nd grade teacher
walk by. I called out to her and asked her
to come join us. I asked what were some
of the things she did to help him focus the
previous year. She explained that she
would sit him next to a student who was
really focused and would reward that
student for reminding my son to look at the

board, or for pointing out what page the class was on. The 3$^{rd}$ grade teacher began to use that intervention.

Another teacher would walk by my son during class and lightly touch his desk if she noticed he was daydreaming. Most teachers used the "usual way" of refocusing our son and would say his name quietly at different times during class. We also discussed with each teacher the importance of him only sitting in the front row but sit in the center. An O.T. student did a study that showed there was a correlation between ADHD and poor eyesight that showed that if a child had to keep turning their head to see the front of the class they would lose focus.

I would also email his teachers when he won an award or had an accomplishment, to help them get to know him as a person outside of their classroom.

# NOTES

# ■QUESTIONS FROM PARENTS

## Do sports & martial arts really work?

*Yes. Adding physical activities to your child's daily routine provides a great outlet to expel energy and helps to get oxygen flowing through the body.*

# NOTES

# What can I do as a mother to help?

*You can be an advocate for your child and fight to get those around you to see how important it is to you to address the symptoms without medication. Educate yourself and those involved with your child's life and be as consistent as possible. Also, you can be patient and try to understand how difficult it is to manage these symptoms. Most importantly, continue to let your child know how much you love them.*

# NOTES

# How do you get your child's school on board with using alternative therapies?

*Schedule meetings with the school staff. Talk to the teachers about interventions they can use to assist your child with maintaining focus while in class. Educate them with articles and other information that you may have.*

# NOTES

**It would be interesting to know how the parent's behavior and the in-home environment impacts the issues?**

*A parent who is able to learn more about the child's symptoms and the different treatment interventions will be better prepared to advocate for their child. A parent who is dealing with a lot of stress may not have the energy to focus on their child and may turn to medication as it may seem like the easier solution. Although difficult it's important for parents to take time for themselves and try to engage in some self-care so that they are better able to take care of their children. Chaos breeds chaos. So, if you are in a home where there is no structure and no organized system, it's difficult to be structured and organized. It's important for the entire family to create a lifestyle in which not only the child can function but the family can function as a whole.*

# NOTES

# What side effects should I prepare to experience when taking them off certain medications?

*It is important to speak with the prescribing physician BEFORE terminating any psychotropic medication treatment. They will explain any side effects that may occur.*

# NOTES

## Is diet in and of itself the best way to treat the situation?

*In my experience, I found that the combination of diet, chiropractic care, the structured routine along with school advocacy and self-esteem building all worked together to create the success that we had. However, I do not think we would have had the most impactful results if we hadn't changed his diet.*

# NOTES

Ok this may sound as though I'm being funny but I'm not. I was talking to my dad about attention disorders and he made a comment that we didn't have those number of issues in the past because discipline and structure worked. What impact does discipline have?

*In the early years, we may not have seen so many of these behaviors because people tended to have a healthier diet with less preservatives and food dye.*

*In the last 40 years or so we had those issues they just weren't so widely diagnosed. Some of the kids were labeled bad, slow, unteachable, etc. Many of those kids ended up self-medicating with drugs and alcohol. Other kids who had ADHD symptoms went unnoticed because there wasn't such a strong focus on testing in schools and there were smaller classrooms and teacher's aides to help give individual attention to those who needed it.*

# NOTES

# Kaleb's Thoughts

What I didn't like about the lifestyle change was I couldn't eat the stuff I wanted to eat. I couldn't eat pizza, candy, bread, bread sticks and things like that. But when I followed my diet and after my chiropractic appointments I did feel better. I understood more of what was happening in class. I would focus more and studying was easier. When I ate junk food and stuff like that I would get distracted and I wasn't able to focus. When I ate french fries at lunch I would be distracted the rest of the day but I still ate french fries because they were good. If I were to tell kids what I liked about this lifestyle, I would tell them that I noticed the difference when I changed my diet. I felt more healthy. I felt like I was more agile. If one day my kids have a hard time focusing, I am going to send them to a chiropractor so they can get a detox and change their diet.

# Acknowledgments

Thank you to everyone who encouraged me to write this book and said our story needed to be told.

To those who helped me daily, I appreciate all the love, care, encouraging words and great advice. Thank U!

To all my family and friends who were sounding boards, editors, proof read this over and over again, gave opinions on book titles and book covers and put up with my constant text messages, emails, questions and parenting meltdowns. You are the best village ever!

I'm grateful for the school administrators and teachers who were flexible and cooperative and went above and beyond to accommodate our son without him having to have a diagnosis or be given special education placement.

A special thank you to my husband Kimoji, who not only went along with this very complex lifestyle change, even when initially he wasn't sure it would work, but implemented most of it in the early years. This would not have been possible without you.

And to my sons, Kaleb Xavier and Kaden Joshua, thank you for working with us as we bombarded you with all these interventions. I know it wasn't easy changing your diet and lifestyle.

We know that you will be able to be anything you want to be in this world. We are so proud to be your parents. We love you! And Kaleb you are perfect just the way you are! Stay focused and keep being you. You got this!

# My Bio

"Day by day in every way, I'm getting better and better." This phrase was told to me by a professor while I was in my second year as a social work student. I continue to use it as a foundation as she assists others in planting seeds of change in their lives.

I have been providing mental health services for over 18 years. I earned both my B.A. in Mass Communication and Masters of Social Work from Clark Atlanta University. While interning in school I provided services in two homeless shelters and oversaw a grant for homeless children. Upon returning to my hometown of Los Angeles, CA, I worked in the foster care system, in group home settings and has provided individual, group and family psychotherapy to at-risk-youth and their families. I am now a Licensed Clinical Social Worker who has been certified to provide Continuing Education Units to other mental health professionals through the California Board of Behavioral Sciences.

"It is amazing to see how many people are suffering from treatable disorders and they don't even know it. My goal is to educate as many people as possible to the importance of learning how to maintain good mental health to have good overall health."

I am a member of the National Association of Social Workers and I am registered with the California Board of Behavioral Sciences. I am also a parenting class instructor and have been certified as a sexual assault crisis volunteer through the YWCA. I have experience as an examination coach and consultant to other licensed clinicians. I am currently a clinical supervisor who provides individual and group clinical supervision to Associate Social Workers, Marriage and Family Therapist Interns, and clinical students. I was previously a part-time lecturer for the School of Social Work at Cal State Long Beach and I run a private practice, New Perspectives in Gardena, CA. Most recently, I have become a

certified health coach and have expanded my practice to assist parents of children who have been diagnosed with ADHD, or mood disorders with treating these issues from a holistic approach. For more information about my programs visit my website
www.newperspectivesprograms.com

I am also the creator and CEO of The Nan Washington Global Wellness Foundation, a non-profit which I created in honor of my grandmother Nannetta J. Washington. Our mission is to provide support to non-profit organizations, schools and those in need, in the form of supplies, education on nutrition, physical and mental health. www.nanwashingtonfoundation.com

To have your question answered in my next book, please feel free to email me at newperspectiveskpb@yahoo.com